BEDROOM JUSTICE

BY

OBI ORAKWUE

BEDROOM POLITICS SERIES

BEDROOM JUSTICE

BY OBI ORAKWUE

BEDROOM JUSTICE

BY OBI ORAKWUE

Be Your Dream Press
Imprint of Obrake USA LLC
New York, NY United States of America

Bedroom Justice

Limit of Liability/Disclaimer
Although all the data and information in this book have been put through an undiscriminating and unsentimental sieve of accuracy and reliability of content, the author and publisher of this book are not liable for any disappointment, commercial, incidental and or consequential damages. If required, consult with a professional before employing the ideas, advice and strategies contained in this book.

 Book Designed by Obrake Designs
Library of Congress Cataloging in Publication Data
Orakwue, Obi
Bedroom Justice/Obi Orakwue
Library of Congress Control Number 2012908993
Includes glossary of terms
ISBN 978-1-948735-02-5 - Paperback Edition
ISBN 978-0-9856222-0-6 – E-book Edition
Printed in USA
First Published in USA in 2012, in E-Book Edition
By Be Your Dream Press
Imprint of Obrake USA LLC
New York, United States of America
www.obrake.com

Dedication

This book is dedicated to natural remedies to imperfection, aging and time, and to all the people who aspire to be armed with knowledge to improve their sex drive, enhance their libido and intensify their orgasm, perfecting their sexual pleasure and optimizing their sex life without appointments and or prescriptions.

Acknowledgments

Thanks to all the people who were involved through research and or interview during the course of writing this book.

TABLE OF CONTENTS

Author's Note 13

Introduction 15

PART 1 17

ATTRACTION: CONTAGION: PHEROMONES:
SYMPATHETIC SCIENCE

CHAPTER 1 18

Optimum Dose of Sex

Conditions/Due Process For Bedroom Justice 19

Attraction

Law attraction

Law of contagion

Pheromones- Chemical Attraction

Positive Mental Attitude

Sex Drive::Libido::Sexual::Desire::Sexual Arousal

Sexual Health and Well-being

Vaginal Muscle Exercise

Optimum Sex Intervals

CHAPTER 2 20

Attraction

The Law of Attraction

The Law of Contagion

CHAPTER 3 24

Pheromones – Chemical Attraction

Pheromones in Other Animals and Plants:...........28

How They May Relate to Humans........................28

PART 2 33

POSITIVE MENTAL ATTITUDE

NON-VERBAL ATTITUDE

CHAPTER 4 35

Positive Mental Attitude

Sympathetic Science/Logic

Factors That May Affect Affectionate/Amorous Memory
Retrieval

Emotional Regulation/Control 39

Creating Amorous Memories 40

PART 3 41

SEXUAL DESIRE AND LIBIDO

CHAPTER 5 42

**SEX DRIVE: LIBIDO: SEXUAL DESIRE: SEXUAL
AROUSAL**

Sex Drive/Libido as an Instinct 42

Dissecting Sex 45

Find Out What You Really Love About Sex: 45

Awaken it

Sight or Visuals

Sound

Environment/Place

Touching

Massage

Exercise

Odor

Taste

Stories

CHAPTER 6 ....**50**

Dissect and Review Your Life

Time Management

How Sleep Affects Your Libido 51

Self-Esteem

CHAPTER 7 ....**54**

 Transforming Your Erotic or Sexual Imagination

And Fantasy into Sexual Desire and Sexual Arousal

Play with Yourself

CHAPTER 8 ....**59**

Vitamins-Minerals for Sexual Desire: Sexual Arousal

Vitamin E

Topical Application of Vitamin E Oil

Vitamin A

Elastin

Collagen

Vitamin C

Vitamin D

VitaminB6

Vitamin K

Minerals for Sex Drive and Libido 64

Magnesium

Selenium

Boron

Manganese

Zinc

Copper

PART 4 67

SEXUAL HEALTH AND WELLBEING

CHAPTER 9 68

Sexual Health and Wellbeing

Dyspareunia

Symptoms of Dyspareunia in Women 70

Causes of Dyspareunia

Natural Causes of Dyspareunia

Acquired Causes of Dyspareunia Include

Dyspareunia in Men

Causes Dyspareunia in Men

Treatment of Dyspareunia in Women

Treatment of Dyspareunia in Men

Interstitial Cystitis

Treatment for Interstitial Cystitis

Peronei's Disease

Urethritis

Prevention

CHAPTER 10 77

SEXUAL DESIRE DISORDER:

SEXUAL AROUSAL DISORDER

Sexual Desire Disorder

Hypoactive Sexual Desire Disorder-HSDD 78

Sexual Aversion Disorder

CHAPTER 11 79

Orgasm (Sexual Gratification)

Orgasm Disorders or Anorgasmia

Types of Anorgasmia

PART 5 83

VAGINAL MUSCLE EXERCISE

CHAPTER 12 84

Vaginal Tightening

Vaginal Muscle Exercise

Kegels Exercise

Identifying the PC Muscle 89

Position to Employ While Exercising-

With Kegel Balls/Devices

Exercise for The Pelvic Floor Muscles..................119

Perineal Massage

Squatting Exercise

PART 6 95

NEUROTRANSMITTERS: ENDORPHINS:

VASODILATORS

CHAPTER 13 96

Bedroom Justice

Neurotransmitters: Endorphins: Vasodilators

Neurotransmitters 97

Endorphins

Vasodilation/Vaso-Dilators

CHAPTER 14...**104**

Innate Style: Sex Accessories: Intervals

General Brief 106

Glossary of Terms 107

About Be Your Dream Press 112

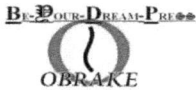

Be-Your-Dream-Press

OBRAKE

Bedroom Justice

Author's Note

The politics of the Bedroom is complex and the most essential politics of any relationship. And the most essential of bedroom politics is bedroom justice; as with anything in human life, being just is often good with no adverse side effect whatsoever. However, as complex and intricate as bedroom politics may be, it has one magic key. The only logical justice in the bedroom is Optimum Dose of Sex – and this can only be attained by healthy and vibrant sex drive, sexual desire, sexual arousal, libido, sexual intercourse and sexual gratification – Orgasm. Once you have healthy libido and sex drive, you have logic and with healthy logic you obtain Justice, in this sense, Bedroom Justice – Optimum Dose of Sex. Sex is very essential to any relationship, it is important to sustain a relationship. Once the sex life of a couple is healthy and enjoyable, other existential problems of a relationship may become more easily managed. However, to have a healthy sexual relationship, you need to have the healthy dose of sex.

Healthy sex drive, libido and ultimately Optimum Dose of Sex may be just a grocery store away. Most active ingredients for the pills for sex drive, sexual desire, sexual arousal and libido are derived from the food, vegetables and plants you see every day. However, you need to know them and know how to eat and employ them to your benefit. All the points, methods, techniques, foods, vitamins and minerals outlined in this book are not quick fix. Maintaining a healthy and mindful lifestyle and incorporating the foods, herbs and exercise discussed in this edition of the book, in your daily way of life should be a primary focus. The understanding that it is a continuous course of duty and lifestyle will make the intake of these foods, herbs, vitamins, minerals and regimen to be effective in increasing and maintaining your sexual health. For best result, articulate daily feeding with doing supplement and vitamins. Some of the herbs are better used on intermittent rather than on a daily basis. Again, as said earlier, the methods and techniques are not any quick fix.

However, some foods, herbs, vitamins and juices are better taken hours and minutes before any bedroom session. It is good to note that mere sexual intercourse and ejaculation is not orgasm and as such does not represent a healthy dose of sex. As you read through the pages of the book, you will see why and how.

Bedroom Justice

INTRODUCTION

For all sexual purposes, the definition of Bedroom Justice points to one thing: Optimum Dose Sex.

Readers are hereby reminded that mere sexual intercourse and ejaculation(s) does not necessarily mean orgasm. Orgasm is rather an intense feeling of relief with the attendant physical and emotional release and surrender to the cellular level of the entire body system. It is the kind of relief and surrender that endures, when you feel you are about to explode with ecstasy: when almost all the cells and tissues of your body system indulge in the said surrender and release of heightened sexual energy in exchange for the ensuing ecstatic explosion.

And that is called Bedroom Justice: Optimum Dose of Sex/Ecstasy.

The steps to achieve this sexual gratification is what will be laid out in the pages of this edition of the book. It is just true that without bedroom Justice, all logic of a relationship, domestic politics and Bedroom politics will be lost. Any and all factors that may inhibit you from having a perfect dose of sex and sexual gratification are trashed out in the pages of this book.

Yes you can still go to paradise with your partner in this lifetime – this guide tells you how and why. All the points, methods, techniques, food, vitamins, minerals and supplements outlined in this book are not quick fix. Maintaining a healthy and mindful lifestyle and incorporating the foods, vitamins, supplements,

Bedroom Justice

exercise and sympathetic science/logic discussed in this edition of the book, in your daily way of life should be a primary focus. The understanding that it is a continuous course of duty and lifestyle will make the intake of these food, supplement, vitamins and minerals to be effective in increasing and maintaining your sexual health and delivering Bedroom Justice to you and your partner. You need to pay attention to all points discussed in this book. When you fail to establish justice in your bedroom, it also affects all aspect of your relationship and ensures Bedroom boredom. Good news is that there is therapy for Bedroom Justice and you can be your own therapist, no prescriptions needed. This guide tells you how.

PART 1

ATTRACTION

CONTAGION

PHEROMONES

SYNPATHETIC SCIENCE

BJ

CHAPTER 1

There is only one logical justice that could be dished out within the confines of the bedroom and within the limits of bedroom politics and bedroom justice. The notable justice is:

- ❖ Optimum Dose of Sex

Once the justice of the bedroom is established, sleep and <u>Optimum Dose of Sleep</u> is better consummated. Sleep is another bedroom justice that needs to be observed with utmost care.

In life, the above duo is hard to overgrow. In other words you can never outgrow sex and sleep. In general, justice of all types whether bedroom or court room justice requires due process, probity, clarity, fairness and relevance to be pronounced/dished out. And in this process there is no partiality.

Optimum dose of sex and optimum dose of sleep could be dependent or correlated to each other. That means it may be difficult to achieve one in total or near absence of the other. A single man or woman may be able to manage and or juggle one in the absence of the other. However, married couples and or people in a live-in relationship may find it more difficult to achieve one in the absence of the other.

Bedroom Justice

As we know, sex is an inalienable and non-negligible part of any relationship and it is the catalyst of love. No relationship based on love, physical attraction and general attraction can survive in the absence of sex and optimum dose of it.

In general, what goes on in the bedroom in any relationship controls and or has about 60% control of the rest of the relationship. In essence, if there is no justice in the bedroom, rarely will there be justice in the entire relationship.

It is fair to say at this point that bedroom justice is to the eye of the presiding judges. What is justice (optimum dose of sex) in the bedroom may differ from couple to couple. However, in all cases, for any bedroom justice to manifest, certain conditions and due process must be in place.

Conditions/Due Process For Bedroom Justice

Attraction - Law of attraction- you can attract positivity and happiness.

Law of Contagion

Pheromones- Chemical Attraction

Positive Mental Attitude

Sex Drive, Libido, Sexual Desire, Sexual Arousal

Sexual Health and Well-being

Vaginal Muscle Exercise

Established and Innate Style and Sex Accessories (optional)

Optimum Sex Intervals

In the following chapters, we will be dissecting each of the above-mentioned conditions.

BJ

CHAPTER 2

ATTRACTION

Some people may choose to call it charm. Notwithstanding the name you desire to recognize it with, attraction, whether physical, chemical, mental, and spiritual are very important in any long-haul relationship and it is of utmost importance in creating optimum setting for justice in the bedroom and subsequently in the entire relationship. One good thing about attraction is that although it could be elusive, however, it could be created, induced, established, <u>maintained in a continuing course</u> and ultimately controlled.

Undoubtedly, there was a cascade of spark, click, pull, that converged into attraction between you and your spouse/partner and that is why you got together in the first instance. However, the cascade of attraction/charm need to be constantly horned, polished, preserved and sustained in an existing and continuing course. The very attraction that brought you people together in the first day and drew you into a relationship through months and probably years could be domesticated and retained forever. Remember, love just like happiness could be transitory.

However, this transitory nature of love and happiness could be hedged and made to be permanent.

Permanent? Yes, the attraction (love) between you and your partner could be tamed to stay in a continuing transitory course within the relationship - -permanent. This means that though you couldn't change the transitory nature of love, it could stay within the relationship with the option of leaving once you stop feeding it the treats that tames it into the continuing course.

You only need to think positively, plan positively and implement positively to domesticate and retain it.

The Law of Attraction as we know it is the attraction or aggregation of 'likes'. It is though better or popularly explained with metaphysical principles than scientific. The 'likes' may be positive, negative and or numb. In other words, the more positive thinking, attitude and or projection you have towards whatever, the more you will be disposed to have a positive result/return/manifestation. You need to control your thoughts, hedge it with positive actions in other to achieve positive manifestation and also to control and influence thoughts by other people, and in this case your spouse/partner. Now, what actually controls the thoughts and subsequently the actions (reactions) of your spouse/partner are your actions which really sprouted from commands of your thoughts.

The Law of Contagion as we know is rooted in the principles of magical thinking. The principles of magical thinking suggests that once two people or objects have been in contact, that a magical link persists between them until a formal exorcism or some other forms of banishing breaks the non-material bond.

In researching the law of contagion, we used examples from psychics, mediums, sorcerers from all cultures and continents including Africa (Nigeria, Ghana, Ivory Coast, and South Africa), Europe (Switzerland, England, France, and Portugal) South America (Brazil, Bolivia, Argentina, and Guyana), Caribbean Island (Jamaica, Antigua, St Martins, and British Virgin Island-Tortola), and North America (Canada, USA, and Mexico). All of them commonly engage/use or desire to engage/use objects owned and utilized by a subject or supposed subject and or even the photograph or image of the subject to carry out psychometry, clairvoyance and or in séances. It therefore means that law of contagion commands a universal recognition, engagement and or acceptance.

And even in today's environment of political correctness, public figures, righteous figures often abhor any physical contact (like hand-shake), to be seen publicly with defamed and or unpopular figures. And we all see it as just part of politics and public insouciance toward unpopular/defamed people. But, it is simply an unconscious acceptance and observance of the law of contagion. Everyone is unconsciously trying to avoid the magical link that may linger once a form of contact is established, whether this is true or not is irrelevant in this observation.

Bedroom Justice

By the same standard, people are often proud to talk about a meeting they had with popular, well-liked, famous, powerful and or holy figures in the society. Some people will proudly display as trophy, a photograph, they snapped with such figures in their offices and living rooms. Figures such as presidents, sports stars, musical icons, popes, movie stars, great writers, etc.

Now how does this observation relate to bedroom justice? Well, it concerns it in the sense that once you have physical and extended physical contacts with a person, a spouse/partner in this case, you can domesticate and control the forces of attraction that brought you together in the first instance. And this is very true when the person is still within touching and physical range. We will go further in explaining contagion using pheromones – chemical attraction.

BJ

CHAPTER 3

PHEROMONES: - CHEMICAL ATTRACTION

The term "pheromone" was introduced by Peter Larlson and Martin Luscher in the year 1959. Pheromone was derived from the Greek word pherein or phero which means to transport, ferry or to bear respectively and the word hormone which means stimulate, stir or arouse. Pheromones are sometimes called ecto-hormones.

Pheromones are chemical factors secreted by an individual and can act, radiate, emit from the body of the secreting/emitting individual to influence the behavior of the receiving individual of the same species. Men release pheromones in their sweat mainly the armpit/underarm sweat. Women release their pheromones when they become fertile. The sensory receptors (vomeronasal organ (VNO) in the olfactory lobes detect the pheromones and send the message to the hypothalamus of the brain for processing. The message triggers sexual desire/arousal and attraction in both sexes. Positive response and invitation depends on the strength of the pheromones and how much the receiving individual is smitten.

Bedroom Justice

It is noteworthy at this point to remember that histamine as we know aids the release of testosterone, the sex drive hormone. Histamine is released by cell bodies (neurons) called histaminergics which is located at the back of the hypothalamus. Histamine is released as a neurotransmitter in the brain.

Remember the love hormone – Oxytocin (discussed in Bedroom Logic and Bedroom Wisdom)? It peaks in the brain and body system during orgasm. Oxytocin is manufactured in the hypothalamus and stored in the thyroid gland. Looks like histamine and oxytocin works very closely.

Tyrosine aids (a precursor) the production of dopamine. Dopamine is an endorphin (endogenous morphine), a feel-good hormone. Tyrosine is processed/produced in the thyroid region, thyroid gland and hypothalamus.

Now, pheromones are processed in the hypothalamus, and its effect will depend on the strength of the particular pheromones to trigger the release of any or the entire thyroid associated endorphins and or their complexes.

These chemicals called Pheromones are capable of acting and only acts outside the body of the secreting individual to impact the behavior of the receiving individual.

It is produced through complex biochemical pathways that the secreting individual is not conscious of. In humans, sex pheromones act as a sex attractant and or trigger mere presence of an opposite sex. Pheromones are received via the sense of smell. The sense of smell is naturally very closely associated with romance, sex drive, sexual desire and sex of the animal kingdom. This makes me remember the he/male goat.

The smell emitted by the opposite sex is a great turn on, sexually. Provided the sensory receptors in the vomeronasal organ (VNO) of the olfactory lobes are healthy, they will transmit the message to the frontal lobe of the brain for processing, and probably ignite/awaken sexual desire and arousal.

Pheromones may elicit/trigger sexual arousal/attraction from a particular individual and trigger mere presence of an opposite sex from another individual, without eliciting any sexual arousal/pull. In essence, pheromones released by say Mr. John may trigger sexual arousal from Ms. Agnes and on the other hand trigger numb (mere presence) from Ms. Jane. It then means that there are receptor sites in the receiving hormones of the females and or males that exhibit friendly reception to the incoming chemical stimuli and trigger sexual desire/arousal and at other times exhibit numb or not-too-friendly reception to the incoming chemical stimuli (pheromones) and trigger no-desire/arousal in the recipient individual.

The difference in the response of receiving individuals has also been explain as the difference in the strength of the pheromones secreted and emitted by individuals as well as the saturation point of the receptor sites of the receiving individuals.

Bedroom Justice

This therefore is not far and or different from the popular saying: "Beauty is to the eye of the beholder". This saying is a lay man's explanation of the existence of natural custom-made attraction be it chemical attraction (pheromones) or otherwise.

And this gives credence to the fact that people by visual examination are attracted to each other because their appearances fit the pattern that is woven through their brains/minds, their own peculiar ideas of a beautiful and attractive person.

By the same standard, the pheromones emitted by people find their fits in the internal hormonal receptor sites of the receiving individual.

This therefore is a form of contagion and attraction.

In this sense, one can be confident in saying that the law of contagion and attraction therefore is not rooted in metaphysical/magical principles, but rather it is rooted in complex biochemical pathways and principles. This complex biochemical pathways and principles may represent magic to a lay mind. Therefore, the term you choose to represent this existential reality is merely semantic.

It is unfortunate that the human sexual chemical pull is mixed with the not-so good armpit sweat. And in today's world of hygiene correctness, it is very rear to find a person that does not use armpit anti-perspirant. Anti-perspirants in the market today are known to block the sweat ducts under the armpit and stops sweating, and in so doing blocks the pheromones from coming out and exerting its effect. Human pheromones are available in the cosmetic and perfume stores, but questions to their efficacy abounds.

Now could that be the reason why it abounds today that so many people are in purportedly love-laden relationships which in reality is only material driven. And as such achieving real amorous bonding becomes difficult, though people can always fake love and attraction. In such situations, bedroom justice and optimum dose of sex is unattainable, recalling that justice of this nature is real and cannot be faked. Remember, mere sexual intercourse and ejaculation does not in itself represent orgasm and optimum dose of sex. – We will discuss this in full detail towards the end (last chapters) of this book.

The question now is: How do you domesticate and control the attraction, chemical attraction and contagion into a continuing and lasting sexual pull?

Simple! Just stay tuned and read on.

Pheromones in Other Animals and Plants:

How They May Relate to Humans

Alarm Pheromones

These types of pheromones are released when insects such as bees, ants and termites are attacked. The pheromones trigger flight in members of same species. Example is when you disrupt with a pen, paper or anything, the order or line of social insects such as ants moving in a single or near single file. What you will observe is a helter-skelter, to-fro, disorderly scuttles of the ants down the formerly organized line of march. This disorganized and apparently disoriented scuttle of the ants is not actually from disorientation from their course of march but because the very group of ants who were at the point of disruption from the pen or paper perceived it as an attack and sent out chemical messages which is received by other member ants who will react or reacted accordingly. If you wait for some 2 to 3 minutes without any further disruption, you will observe the ants regroup and continue in their organized single file line. At this point some trail pheromones may have been released suggesting no-more danger and they continue in their original course. We will discuss trail pheromones as you read further. Plants release these types of pheromones when grazed on by plant eating animals (herbivores). The surrounding plants are then notified of an enemy, and they respond by releasing tannins. Tannins are bitter tasting and less palatable to the offending grazer.

Epideictic Pheromones

These types of pheromones are used by egg laying insects to advise other insects intending to lay eggs in the vicinity and or in the very spot, to find another spot because they (pheromones emitting insect) have taken position in the space in question. These pheromones must not be mistaken for territorial pheromones.

Releaser Pheromones: These pheromones trigger quick response from the targets. However, they have short efficacy span. These pheromones attract members of same species from afar.

Signal Pheromones

Chemical signals from theses pheromones trigger short-term changes and responses.

Primer Pheromones

Chemicals from primer pheromones often exert a very slow trigger, however, the duration of the effect lasts very long once started. The effect of primer pheromones are often towards a developmental change. In mammals, it is believed that nursing mothers secret and emits this chemical molecule (mammary pheromones) to trigger nursing behavior in their babies. Mammals such as rabbits, dogs, cats, sheep and goats secrete and emit these chemical molecules. It has been said that when a new born refuse to suckle or breast feed, it is because the mother didn't and couldn't emit these pheromones to trigger the primer.

Territorial Pheromones

Mammals such as dogs, cats, monkeys, chimps use this type of pheromones to carve out territorial perimeter and control.

Birds also has been shown to use territorial pheromones, as found in social birds that use their preen glands secretion to mark their nests and love/marital/nuptial gifts.

Trail Pheromones

These types of pheromones are used by social insects to mark their paths to serve as guide to and from their holes. It has also been suggested to be the pheromones which lost dogs use to find their way home, and or find their peers way from their comfort territory. These types of pheromones are also used by ants. Remember the ants when they ferry particles into their ant hole and trace their way back to the food resource point to fetch some more particles.

Sex Pheromones

Sex pheromones in animals are used identify the availability of the female for breeding.

Farmers use sex pheromones to detect fertility readiness (oestrus) in female pigs (sows). In doing this, the farmers will spread Male pig (Boar) pheromones in the pig pen (sty) and any female (sow) that has oestrus or ready for breeding will automatically be sexually aroused.

Appeasement Pheromones

These types of pheromones have been identified in mammals. It is use to calm situations and aggressive approach.

***** *****

In general, mammals' pheromones are detected primarily by the vomeronasal organ (VNO). Vomeronasal organ (VNO) is chemosensory organ located at the base of the nasal septum. An active role for the human VNO in the detection of pheromones is still being disputed by some scientists. The VNO in developing fetuses has been demonstrated. However, the VNO are found to be greatly diminished into membranes in adults. The pheromone receptors in the human vomeronasal organ are V1Rs, V2Rs and V3Rs, and they are all G protein-coupled receptors. They are also found to be somehow related to the common receptors in the olfactory system. Their distant resemblance to the main olfactory receptors identifies their separate or different function in the sense of smell family.

It is a well-known fact that courteous behaviors such as smile, greeting and compassion are contagious. By the same standard, hostile and not-so-courteous thoughts will also be contagious. The contagion may result from a developed chemical pathway in the subjects in play. It is therefore inferred that one's thinking, and behavior as regards the bedroom may generate a kind of chemical pathway that may be secreting and emitting some forms of pheromones in response, and the target subject, in this case a spouse/partner will react to the command/effect of the emitted pheromones.

98% of all people interviewed during the course of writing this book responded that seeing or knowing that their spouse/partner is on heat or sexually aroused, turns them on and vice versa. <u>All effects are reflections of their causes.</u>

***** *****

***** *****

PART 2

POSITIVE MENTAL ATTITUDE
NON-VERBAL ATTITUDE

BJ

CHAPTER 4

POSITIVE MENTAL ATTITUDE

The central theme in this psychological coinage is that: You are what you think, but most importantly how you set out to practice what you think. Success may be achieved through practically attainable, deliberate goal-directed and optimistic thoughts and thought process. Now take this to our theory and explanation of the effects of chemical secretions/ emissions, attraction and contagion. All effects are reflections of their causes. Amorous thinking will definitely elicit the secretion of sex pheromones through biochemical pathways and emit such to the partner, and by the same standard, a stressful and hateful thinking will elicit the secretion of alarm/flight/repulsive pheromones and emit such to the partner.

Sympathetic Science/Logic

Different people call it names as they deem best including sympathetic science, sympathetic logic, and sympathetic magic. It is sometimes called imitative science imitative logic or imitative magic. This is a type of science or invocative practice based on imitation, repeat/recall and or correspondence.

Bedroom Justice

Every relationship has a peak and or the so-called honeymoon stage. You can invoke this stage of your relationship through imitation and invocation of re-constructible/repeatable relationship experiences including words, visuals/looks, music, sentences, phrases, dispositions, positioning, revisiting of places or similar places, dressing, grooming and priming. The theory and application of the principles of

sympathetic science is based on two models namely similarity and contagion/contact. As said earlier, effects and causes are similar, equal and opposite.

Now, at this stage, you may be acting years away from the peak /honeymoon era of your relationship. The correspondence or effect of your invocation is simply laid out on the rules of correspondence, in that effect or influence could be triggered due to nostalgic resemblance to the moments of joy and ecstatic peak in the relationship.

By so doing, you will be using circumstantial similarities to induce instincts through emotional stimuli to create essentially the same physiological condition by enhancing the production of neurotransmitters (brain chemicals) that will induce neuro-chemical activity that affects sections of the brain (amygdala) which is responsible for encoding (interpreting) stimuli and retrieving memory, in this case lovable memory. The section of the human brain that interprets stimuli and retrieves memory in this sense is the amygdala. Once the stimuli is strong enough to retrieve the desired memory, the subsequent action will be secretion of endorphins (love or feel-good brain chemicals) in response to the retrieved amorous memory and the ensuing amorous feeling and expression. Does it sound like too much to be doing just for bedroom justice?

Well, may be, however, anything worth having and or enjoying is worth working for. And while you toil to elicit this effect on your spouse/partner, you are triggering it in yourself.

Sympathetic science or logic is what is in play when people buy celebrity collectibles such as a guitar (or even the replica) used by say John Lenon, Bob Marley, Elvis Presley, etc. Another example is when people will want to buy the pen used by say the American President to sign the Bill of Rights or use a copy of the bible used by the dead popular pope, say John Paul. It is somewhat a general notion that the objects/collectibles possess energy of those special people, and the special events. Another example is religious pilgrimages to holy lands of Jerusalem, Mecca and elsewhere.

Now the difference which is a positive difference is that with you and your partner, all subjects present in the desired past period are also present in the present time, thus it is more likely to potentiate the laws of attraction, contagion and sympathetic science.

As said in the paragraph above, the use of emotional stimuli will produce neurotransmitters, neuro-chemical activity and eventually retrieval of memory.

Bedroom Justice

The recalled memory will then trigger arousal which will dwell on different frequencies ranging from calming or soothing to exciting or exhilarating. So, in essence you used similarity and resemblance to elicit emotional enhancement effect on memory which then adjusts through different stages of formation and reconstruction which is called memory arousal phases. The frequency/phase at which the memory settles is dependent on how the memory was stored at the time of the experience.

At the stage of memory arousal, sexual desire and sexual arousal becomes far easier and completely attainable if the subjects are sexually healthy. However, with time and repeats of emotional stimuli, and ensuing memory arousal, delays may be experienced before effective memory arousal is achieved and the delay will be incremental albeit slowly with time and subsequent repeats of the same circumstantial similarities and resemblances. This diminishing response in arousal is explained from the fact that frequent repeat of levels of memory arousal from the same emotional stimuli using the same circumstantial similarity and nostalgic resemblance will lead to narrowing or decrease in sensitivity towards the stimuli due to probable saturation of the neural receptor sites. In lay words it may lead to routine. To avoid this, you must use different circumstantial similarities and resemblances at each session and repeat of sessions must be far between. At other times, you may want to mix and match different circumstantial similarities and resemblance to create a cascade of emotional stimuli and memory arousal.

Mix and match have been shown to produce a fast and strong sexual desire and sexual arousal. This may be because of stronger secretion of neurotransmitters and endorphins into the nervous system. What was not clear is whether different neurotransmitters and endorphins were secreted into the nervous system in response to the different segments of the mixes and matches. It is good to note that the present/current mood of the subject(s) will also influence the retrieval of past experiences and memories. At this point, we have established that there are joyful and retrievable love and affectionate memories of the relationship that is permanently embedded in our conscious and subconscious minds.

Now domesticating and controlling these loveable and good memories of past experiences is nothing more than retrieving the said experiences using circumstantial similarities and resemblances. It is pertinent to create more of the experiences even as we retrieve the past ones.

Therefore, perfecting the art of desirable memory retrieval with regards to spousal, nuptial, amorous and significant-other relationships is essential to attaining bedroom justice. And nobody should know better how to retrieve and induce emotional stimuli to trigger memory arousal and ensuing sexual desire and sexual arousal in your spouse/partner more than you and this assertion is in line with the no-partiality streak of due process of bedroom justice and justice in general.

Factors That May Affect: -

Affectionate/Amorous Memory Retrieval

The present/current mood of the subject (partner): - the present mood of your partner may influence the retrieval of your past affectionate memories. The current mood may cause the emotional stimuli to elicit a rapid/quicker and or slower memory arousal as the case may be.

Emotional Regulation/Control

It has been shown that efforts to regulate or control emotion at the time it was created/formatted may be a factor in retrieving the experience and how the emotional stimuli will affect the memory arousal. If there wasn't enough emotional expression at the time the experience was created, and the memory stored, it is possible that during retrieval, the memory arousal will be weak. In essence what this is saying is that in love and relationship matters, it is very essential to completely surrender to the ecstasy of the experience and be emotionally expressive, because suppressing or regulating your emotion will inevitably affect and undermine the memory of such experience. And this will form part of the memory of the experience.

CREATING AMOROUS MEMORIES

Now that you have learnt the essence and application of sympathetic science or sympathetic logic, there is no doubt that you may have identified the necessity of creating memorable experiences that may be retrieved in the future for purposes of optimizing your love life and bedroom justice. In creating memorable experiences, you will be priming your partner into a continuing amorous relation with you through priming, using affectionate and erotic interaction, presentation, dinning, words, dance, music and outing/outdoors events. The more you prime your partner, the better the response of a future experience and stimuli, until you get to the level of Pygmalion effect. Pygmalion effect states that the more and better you treat people, the better they will perform in the future. Noting that the difference between a queen and a plebian woman lies more on how they are treated. It is therefore pertinent that in creating an amorous experience, you need to get a little creative; after all, you are only giving yourselves treats. And what is better in creativity than the creativity directed towards one's consumption/utilization.

***** *****

PART 3

SEXUAL DESIRE AND LIBIDO

***** *****

***** *****

BJ

CHAPTER 5

SEX DRIVE: LIBIDO: SEXUAL DESIRE: SEXUAL AROUSAL

For Bedroom Justice (optimum dose of sex) to be attained, one needs first of all to have sexual desire and sexual arousal, without sexual desire and arousal, sexual intercourse may not be consummated. In this chapter, we will discuss sex drive and sexual arousal with regards to optimum dose of sex, however, more details on Sex Drive and Libido is completely laid out in the book: The Bedroom Logic.

As discussed from chapter one through chapter 4, the due process for bedroom justice needs to be in place and complete for optimum dose of sex which is the ultimate of bedroom justice. And in continuing to awaken and institute the due process, we will now discuss libido awakening/reawakening.

SEX DRIVE/LIBIDO IS AN INSTINCT

Sex Drive and Libido is inherent to humans and has components that are delicately interwoven and connected since birth. Sometimes it is at its normal energetic level (during certain ages of life) or it may lie low (sleeping) and needs some awakening.

And at other times it may be bruised and needs some revival, or it may be dead/damaged and needs to be remedied. Notwithstanding the state of the human sex drive, it is always possible to rekindle libido.

Yes You Can Still Have Sex Again and have optimum dose of sex in this Lifetime!

For the purpose of this chapter, let's divide Sex Drive into three Components:

- ❖ Imagination/Fantasy/Dream
- ❖ Urge – renewable inherent energy encased in the subconscious
- ❖ Sex and Orgasm - release and surrender of the renewable energy

The imagination, fantasy or dream is driven and directed by the trapped inherent renewable subconscious sexual energy. The urge to reach out for the physical contact or consummation of the fantasy/imagination is driven by hormones.

The awakening of this energy to drive the imagination, fantasy or desire is the process of bringing it up from the subconscious to the conscious level, and the process differs from one individual to another. The process is always as diverse as the cause of the 'sleep', (libido sleep) which may range from emotional, psychological, physical, etc., as discussed in the previous book "Bedroom Logic" under causes of Low Libido/Sex Drive.

Bedroom Justice

Remember, the energy of sex, the energy of sexual desire and attraction to the opposite sex is not an ordinary or banal energy. It is the energy of the continuity of life, and in this case, the energy is an integral component of the chemistry of the continuity of human existence. And this energy is alive throughout life even when what we know within the realms of biological possibility points to the contrary. It could be awakened and revived at any point of human life.

At a certain stage in life, one wouldn't necessarily need to have sex with another human being (sexual intercourse) to be and feel sexed. At that and such points, it is not so much as having interest in physical sexual intercourse as in being able to articulate the entire sexual energy, including erotic energy, nervous system energy, the endocrine system energy, sensory system energy, the lymphatic system energy, the digestive system energy, visual energy, emotional energy into that awakening and enlightening pull.

It is just very true that nothing awakens and enlightens the brain and the entire body system more than the pull of sexual attraction and desire.

To have a smooth and effective reawakening of sex drive, we need to dissect sex into its entire components and then identify the part(s) that most turns us on. And once you identify what is your softest spot of sex and sexual desire, then you can conveniently work on it, to unleash the energy.

In working on the most erotic stimuli of your sexual imagination and fantasy, you must surrender, and block away all and any inhibition that may block your freedom of imagination and fantasy.

DISSECTING SEX:
FIND OUT WHAT YOU REALLY LOVE ABOUT IT AND AWAKEN IT

SIGHT OR VISUALS

Visualizing/seeing a potential sex partner is the first step and feeling you endure of sexual attraction. Even in your imagination and dreams of sexual fantasy, there is always a picture of the type of sexual partner that is interwoven into your psyche of what an attractive partner should look like. The magic of visual conception and fascination is an integral part of sex drive and sexual energy. To awaken your sex drive, you need to rekindle this pictorial imagination and fantasy by visiting and or positioning yourself where it is most possible to see your type (physical) of partners. You may need to visit places for this purpose. The beaches, downtown, parks, gardens, schools, movie theaters, rallies, concerts, all places you may see a variety of people, etc., are good places to start.

SOUND

There are sounds associated with some intimate and romantic moments of your sexual life. Sounds that make your sex drive boom and boost. Such sounds form part of the entire sexual desire and drive. Reintegrating yourself with such sounds will add a positive forward step to the awakening process of your sex drive.

Sounds Such As:

- ✓ Music
- ✓ Melody
- ✓ Singing birds
- ✓ Roaring tide
- ✓ Stream
- ✓ The creek
- ✓ Moaning
- ✓ Laughter
- ✓ Wind

ENVIRONMENT/PLACE

Certain types of environment and place evoke sexual desire in people. It may be some quiet place in the woods, by the banks of a lonely and quiet river/creek, the beach, the theater, sand-dooms, mountain, valleys, hilly country side, the sea, etc.

TOUCHING

Touch for the most part could be erotic and stirs sexual desire. If touching is one of the acts that stir your sex drive, then you need to employ it. The touching could be massage by a professional masseur or touching from your sex partner. Whichever one that floats your boat is the one you need to employ. Always remember the hugs, those little goodbye hugs to your partner, it works like magic.

MASSAGE

As explained in the book 'The Bedroom Logic' touch and hug enhance the release of oxytocin. Using that standard, Oxytocin therefore can be released by various types of sensory stimulation including massage. Bloodstream levels of oxytocin have been shown to rise during massage. Oxytocin is a love hormone.

EXERCISE

Exercise brings the release of endorphins and also wards off depression. Some exercise has been touted to induce labour; the hormone oxytocin is abundant in the body system of delivering mothers. By that standard, it is possible that exercise may help to induce the secretion of oxytocin in normal non-pregnant males and females. Exercise also induces the secretion of other endorphins including dopamine, the feel-good hormone.

ODOR

The sense of smell is naturally very closely associated with romance, sex drive, sexual desire and sex of the animal kingdom. Remember the he goat?

The smell emitted by the opposite sex is a great turn on, sexually. Provided the sensory receptors in the vomeronasal of the olfactory lobes are healthy, they will transmit the message to the frontal lobe of the brain for processing, and probably ignite/awaken sexual desire. See chapter 3 – Chemical Attraction

Bedroom Justice

TASTE

Taste is an integral part of the sensory system and plays a role in awakening sex drive and or sexual desire. Some people's sexual desire and or drive may be associated with a particular taste. It may be taste of food, fruit, drink and or the taste of kissing.

You know more than anybody else what floats your boat. Employ it to your sex drive awakening process.

STORIES

Nothing creates and revives imagination and fantasies more than stories.

Such stories include:

Printed Stories with images and pictures- Pictorials, Sex magazines

Printed stories – romance novels

Visual Stories – Movies, sex films

If this is what floats your sex imagination boat, then indulge in it. In doing all that is outlined in this section of the book, you need not rush. You must continue with dissecting and re-dissecting sex until you find the real thing that floats your sexual imagination and fantasy. Once you find it or them, you must act on it until you start to have sexual imagination and fantasy again. Do not rush, it is therapy. Once you reawaken your imagination, and sexual fantasy, you are done with the stage.

Bedroom Justice

At this point you have awakened the primary part of sex drive, which is sexual/erotic imagination and fantasy. The next step is to transform the imagination and fantasy into sexual desire

BJ

CHAPTER 6

DISSECT AND REVIEW YOUR LIFE

In the last chapters, we dissected sex and identified what you actually like most about sex, and have you work on them to awaken your libido.

Now, it is only reasonable if we pay attention to the fingers that are pointing back at you while you were pointing the accusing/dissecting finger at sex. We will now have you review your life to see if there is anything within you which is as much a culprit.

What is your daily schedule including from the time you wake up, to the breakfast table, to leaving for work through coming back home to going back to sleep at bed time.

Make a detailed list of it, leaving nothing behind. Do you have enough rest/break time in-between your daily shores? Remember, the body needs consistent break time and rest to restore and replenish energy, minerals and hormones for proper functioning. When the body does not receive enough rest it is stressed out and the stress will start to accumulate in the system, big enemy of libido. When stress accumulates stress hormone (cortisol) is released and it is a big time enemy/inhibitor to sexual desire and sexual arousal.

Do you have enough sleep in every 24-hour cycle of the day? Nothing substitutes sleep, not even rest. Enough sleep is a must for the proper and optimal functioning of all the body system including the nervous system, the endocrine system, the brain, and sensory system, the immune system, reproductive system, the circulatory system, any and all the system of the body is directly or indirectly dependent on sleep for replenishment. Remedy is Simple – Make out more time for relaxation, rest and sleep. You need at least seven hours sleep every 24hours cycle. Of the 7-hour sleep time, 6 hours must be straight sleep preferably during night time. The remaining one hour could be shared between naps during normal daily activity.

No matter how busy you are, you can achieve the 7-hr minimum sleep time every 24hr cycle if you employ proper time management for your schedule

Time-Management

Allot time and limit to all and every of your daily activity. Make out time for rest/break between activities. Make out time for naps between activities. Manage your time adequately, and do not over work yourself.

HOW SLEEP AFFECTS YOUR LIBIDO

Sleep is an elevated restful and anabolic state. During sleep, revival, growth and rejuvenation of the immune, nervous, reproductive, skeletal and muscular systems takes place. It is very important to most members of the animal kingdom including all mammals, all birds, many reptiles, amphibians, and fish. Chemicals called *neurotransmitters* control sleep or wakefulness by acting on different groups of nerve cells, or neurons in the brain. Neurons in the brainstem, which connects the brain with the spinal cord, produce neurotransmitters such as serotonin and norepinephrine. Serotonin and Norepinephrine keep some parts of the brain active while we are awake. A chemical called adenosine accumulates in the blood while we are awake and causes drowsiness if we stay too long without sleep. This chemical gradually breaks down while we sleep. Neurons that control sleep interact closely with the immune system. Decreased serotonin levels can lead to chronic stress and fatigue, sleep disorders and changes in appetite. Fatigue is an enemy of healthy sex drive.

Chronic stress depletes the body of nutrients and destabilizes the optimal stable state of the brain and endocrine system/chemistry. Over-worked sympathetic nervous system leads to chronic stress and a range of adverse condition includes insomnia, adrenal fatigue, restlessness, muscular tension and pain, gastrointestinal problems, and ultimately low sex drive, low libido, low sexual desire and low sexual arousal.

Human Growth Hormone (HGH) is replenished and its level in the body system rises during deep sleep. The human body relies on chemical components to maintain a constant state of balance. This state of balance is called homeostasis. When one or more of the body chemicals fall out of balance due to increase or decrease in their levels, this may cause the systems of the body to work less efficiently. Chemical imbalances in the reproductive system can cause infertility and low Sex Drive in both men and women. Low levels of estrogen and testosterone can affect sex drive, sexual desire and sexual performance.

Self-Esteem

Strong and high self-esteem breeds feel good state of mind. Feeling good and high self-esteem accentuates sensuality and boost sexual drive and sexual desire. Low self-esteem may be due to dissatisfaction with one's appearance including body weight, structure and or shape.

For more information on this topic, please see the Book: **Bedroom Logic**, by Be Your Dream Press.

***** *****

BJ

CHAPTER 7

TRANSFORM EROTIC-SEXUAL IMAGINATION AND FANTASY INTO SEXUAL DESIRE, SEXUAL AROUSAL

Now that the sexual imagination and fantasy have been awakened through dissecting sex and identifying what turns you/your partner on the most, the mind has been awakened and the brain stimulated. The cerebral cortex of the frontal lobe of the brain is the origin of command for the production of physical stimuli – the hormones that drive sexual desire, arousal or urge. The sexual desire and or arousal will be revived in anticipation for sexual activity. In an earlier chapter we made mention of the fact that the amygdala is the part of the brain responsible for producing and giving commands as regards memory arousal from emotional stimuli. At this metamorphic stage of your sexuality and sensuality, you need to reconnect your physical self with the physical erotic stimuli and the sexual imagination. In so doing, you will learn if the sexual imagination and the physical stimuli bring sexual desire and sexual arousal.

Furthermore, you will also learn if the desire and or arousal lead to penile erection in case of men or vaginal lubrication, genital engorgement and in some cases, nipples hardening in case of women.

Remember, as said in the earlier chapters, sex drive is an instinct driven by sexual energy. The energy is encased in the subconscious and the process of awakening your sexual imagination, and transferring it from the mind to the brain, where physical stimuli that drives the energy from the brain through the spinal cord to the S2-S4 sacral nerve is generated.

The energy is delivered to the pelvic splanchnic nerves which start from the sacral spinal nerves S2 to S4 otherwise called Pelvic splanchnic nerves. From here, the energy is dissipated, and they contribute to the innervation/blood supply of the pelvic floor and genital organs, supplying the capillaries in the region. If the above is established, then, you have lifted your sexual energy from the subconscious mind where it was encased to the conscious mind where it is at liberty to unleash.

How Do We Know You Did this?
PLAY WITH YOURSELF

Sounds odd, doesn't it? Somehow, yes. However, it does not really sound proper when playing with oneself becomes odd. In other words, it is embarrassing in itself to know that people feel odd, shy and embarrassed when masturbation is brought up for discussion. Playing with oneself should not necessarily be for orgasm to be achieved, really it is more of sexual/circulatory/innervation exercise to make sure that blood supply and circulation to the genitals is healthy. Practicing this blood circulatory exercise to achieve arousal/erection or engorgement of the genitals is very healthy in itself and may preserve your sexual arousal health. Trying out with yourself is a way of improving the animal instinct of sexuality (sexual desire) in you, if possible increasing it many folds to bring the urge and sexual desire (sex drive) to the level where you will be grabbing or reaching out for the physical contact/consummation of your sexual fantasy/imagination, sexual desire with another human being. If that happens then you have completely reawakened, revived and or remedied your sex drive, your libido. Playing with yourself does not necessarily mean achieving or reaching orgasm, but, merely to see if you can get some arousal. It is a healthy sexual exercise. Remember, the whole process started because you need Bedroom Justice (optimum dose of sex) and you need to put in place due process that will enable you to have your piece of bedroom justice and it includes making sure that even if you have low or diminished sex drive, it will be revived. You are engaged in a therapy. There is this misconception about masturbation. Most people think masturbation is for people who don't have sex partners, but it is not true, at least for the purpose of this book, and this study. Besides, if you don't know how to be sensual and sexual with yourself, if you do not know how to arouse yourself, then, how do you expect to be good at it with a partner? For the purpose of this section of the book, this therapy, you need to try it to see the connection you have made between your sexual fantasy, the erotic stimuli originating from the cerebral cortex of the frontal lobe of the brain and the physical you. Once the three links are connected, and established, your sex drive/libido is revived, and you will then go on to the next stage which is sexual gratification - orgasm.

Tried it?

Did you have erection?

Vaginal Lubrication?

Nipples Hardening?

Yes? Bingo!

No? ooh!

If you do not achieve erection, vaginal lubrication, or if you do have a minimal or weak erection, minimal lubrication, it means that the erotic physical stimuli provided by the hormones are weak and not enough to sustain the imagination and fantasy that have been awakened.

This will take us to Sex Drive Revival through remedies/therapy such as:

- ➢ Food
- ➢ Vitamins
- ➢ Minerals
- ➢ Aphrodisiacs
- ➢ Hormone Replacement
- ➢ Etc.

Bedroom Justice

For complete detail as regards reviving Sex Drive through remedies/therapy using the bulleted points above, please see the book **"The Bedroom Logic"**

In the next chapter we will discuss vitamins and minerals as regards Bedroom Justice - Optimum Dose of Sex. More details could be found in the Book:

The Bedroom Fool.

BJ

CHAPTER 8

VITAMINS: MINERALS FOR SEXUAL DESIRE: SEXUAL AROUSAL

Vitamins and minerals as they affect sexual desire and sexual arousal is well explained in the books:

The Bedroom Fool and Bedroom Logic. We will discuss them sparingly in this section of the book.

In other to have sexual desire, sexual arousal and optimum dose of sex (bedroom Justice), you need to be sexually virile. Sexual virility is well primed with the use of among other things vitamins and minerals. Vitamins provide substances that human body may not be producing due to hormonal imbalance, other nutritional deficiencies and or because they are essential vitamins. Essential vitamins are those vitamins that the body system does not produce on their own, example includes vitamin C.

VITAMIN E

Vitamin E has been said to aid in the production of sex hormones including estrogen, progesterone and testosterone.

Vitamin E oil sometimes called the sex vitamin is helpful for rejuvenating dry vaginal tissues when taken orally and when used as a topical application.

TOPICAL APPLICATION OF VITAMIN E OIL

The topical application of vitamin E oil is mainly for lubrication. Some women use the oil from Vitamin E capsules to replicate vaginal lubrication. Applying Vitamin E oil on a daily basis rehydrates the vaginal tissue. The walls of the vaginal canal incorporate the moisture from vitamin E oil back into its natural processes.

See the Book: - Bedroom Fool for more information.

VITAMIN A

Vitamin A maintains the health of the epithelial tissues which line all the external and internal surfaces of the body, including the linings of the vagina wall and the uterus in women. Vaginal wall consists of stratified squamous epithelial muscles.

Generally, sex hormones including estrogen have DNA receptor sites, and vitamin A is in the family that is friendly to the receptors.

Vitamin A helps in the regulation of the synthesis of the sex hormone, progesterone, which in turn helps in balancing the levels of estrogen and testosterone.

ELASTIN

Elastin or otherwise called tropoelastin is a structural protein responsible for elasticity (stretching, rebound or recoil) found mainly in connective tissues such as vaginal wall, the penis, skin, blood vessels (chiefly the aorta), joints, ligaments, cartilages. Elastin allows tissue to resume or return to their original shape/size after stretching or contracting. In this case, it helps the vagina to return to its original size after stretches such as in child-birth, insertion of large objects, and loosening. In the human body, elastin is biochemically coded by the gene known as the ELN. Elastin is made up of randomly coiled fibers of about 830 essential amino acids that are cross-linked into a durable form, and lysine is chiefly responsible for the cross-linkage. The two types of links found in elastin are: desmosine link and isodesmosine link.

Remember the ridges or folds of the vaginal wall?

Elastin is responsible for the ridges (coils or folds).

Deficiency of elastin causes:

General loss of elasticity such as in blood vessels, Loose vagina, Loose bladder (incontinence)

Elastin therefore aids in the health of the blood vessels, as such it is very essential to adequate and proper blood circulation and supply. Proper blood circulation and supply is a primer to erection, sexual desire, sexual arousal, sex drive and libido and ultimately optimum dose of sex.

COLLAGEN

Collagen like elastin is commonly found in penile tissues, vaginal muscles, connective tissues such as ligaments, blood vessels, skin, bones, lungs, eye (cornea) and gut in the form of elongated fibril (strands of fibrillin -glycoproteins). Collagen is created in the body cells called fibroblast. Collagen and elastin work in coordination to maintain the elasticity of the vagina and penile tissues.

VITAMIN C

Vitamin C is involved in the synthesis of sex hormones such as androgen, estrogen and progesterone. Vitamin C helps to increase libido and also highly effective in increasing fertility. Vitamin C is essential for the production of collagen and elastin, both forms part of the support to the vaginal attachment to the pelvic floor. Collagen and elastin also forms part of the penis muscular fibers and responsible for penile stretching and recoil. Elastin is the structural protein responsible for the elasticity of the vagina, the vaginal wall and vaginal canal.

VITAMIN D

Vitamin D is an essential part of the endocrine system. Vitamin D helps to regulate several of the adrenal hormones, growth of cells, and production of enzymes. DHEA is produced by the adrenal glands. DHEA or Dehydroepiandrosterone is a steroid hormone produced by the body to create both male and female hormones. DHEA is secreted naturally in the body by the adrenal glands. DHEA and estrogen hormone levels in the body tends to peak in the twenties and decline as people get older. DHEA is converted in the body to both the female hormone, estrogen and the male hormone testosterone.

VITAMIN B6

Vitamin B6 is necessary for metabolism of protein, fat and amino acids, hormonal function (estrogen and testosterone), and the production of red blood cells, and neurotransmitters (serotonin, norepinephrine, dopamine, GABA –gama-aminobutyric acid). GABA is directly responsible for the regulation of muscle tone including smooth muscles such as vaginal and pc muscles. Vitamin B6 is essential for the general good of the nervous system. It is very important for keeping stress away.

Vitamin B6 is directly involved in synthesis and secretion of dopamine in the brain, dopamine gives a feel-good mood. Feel-good mood is love mood and sex drive friendly.

Vitamin B6 is essential for conversion of selenium in its dietary state (selenomethionine) into an absorbable form by the body.

Vitamin B6 helps in controlling elevated prolactin and in so doing functions as a libido enhancer. Vitamin B6 helps to balance the levels of progesterone and estrogen. Ingesting Vitamin B6 regularly, helps a woman reach orgasm and sometimes increases sexual stamina of both men and women.

VITAMIN K

Vitamin K is very good for blood circulation in the capillaries and general capillary health. The blood circulatory function of vitamin K aids adequate blood innervation of the capillaries in the genital region. Blood supply to the genitals is good for sexual desire, sexual arousal, erection and general sex drive and libido.

***** *****

MINERALS FOR SEX DRIVE AND LIBIDO

MAGNESIUM

Magnesium is essential for energy metabolism, proper functioning of the muscle in the body system including vaginal wall muscles, pelvic floor muscles and penile muscles. Magnesium is also good for nerve functions, and formation of cell membranes. Magnesium is also essential in the production of sex hormones like androgen, estrogen and neurotransmitters (dopamine and norepinephrine) that regulates libido. Magnesium supplements are available over the counter from the drug stores

SELENIUM

Selenium is vital to ensure the production of healthy ova & sperms. It acts as a coenzyme to calcium and magnesium. Selenium assists sperm production and also aid sperm motility. Selenium is most abundantly situated in the seminal ducts and the testes.

Selenium supplement is available over the counter in drug stores.

BORON

Boron is a trace mineral/element, which means its body daily need is small. Boron can influence the production and estrogen metabolism in the body system. Boron increases levels of estrogen in women and testosterone in men. It is used to help regulate sex hormones, especially in women going through menopause, and diminishes the need for Hormone replacement therapy (HRT). While boron supplement works well for some women, it may worsen menopausal symptoms in some other women. Boron regimen in premenopausal, menopausal and postmenopausal women presents fast result in improved sex drive, libido and vaginal lubrication. Symptom of menopause such as hot flashes and depression were quickly eliminated in women undergoing boron regimen. One can overdose on supplemental boron. Boron could become toxic in high doses. Use with care. Boron supplement is available over the counter in your neighborhood drug stores.

MANGANESE

Manganese is essential for the synthesis of fatty acids, which is necessary for a healthy nervous system. The nervous system is somewhat the electrical system of the body. The nervous system regulates the production and secretion of hormones.

ZINC

The Zinc is good for the production of testosterone, the sex hormone that boosts sexual desire, sexual arousal, sex drive and libido in both men and women. Zinc in combination with B vitamins is excellent for sperm count (semen volume) and fertility. Healthy zinc level in the body is same as healthy testosterone level in the body. Healthy testosterone level in the body (male and female) means high sex drive or high libido.

Zinc in combination with B6 and B9 (folate/folic acid) raises sperm production, sperm count (semen volume) and testosterone production. Low levels of zinc in the body system have been since linked to poor libido in men and women. Zinc in combination with Vitamin B6 + Vitamin B9 + Selenium is very good for the good quality sperm production including sperm count/quantity/volume, sperm motility, sperm viability and virility.

COPPER

Copper has healing properties. Copper in conjunction with Vitamin C and Zinc provides and environment for the optimal production of elastin and elastin fibers. Increase intake of Zinc requires increased intake of copper. Copper is deeply involved in the electrical and transportation system of the body. Elastin and collagen are essential for the health and optimal functioning of vaginal muscle and penile fiber and muscle.

***** *****

PART 4

SEXUAL HEALTH AND WELLBEING

BJ

CHAPTER 9

SEXUAL HEALTH AND WELLBEING

The commonest culprit for sexual injustice and inadequate dose of sex is the fear and reluctance to engage in sexual activity. Most people are very reluctant to engage in penetrative sex and any form of sex whatsoever because they are afraid of discomfort associated with sexual intercourse, which is often caused by sexual unhealthiness. Sexual unhealthiness may bring a feeling of shame, inadequacy and feeling or fear of being inadequate, unfit, and defective on the act and this can be highly troubling.

Such lapses in sexual health and wellbeing may include the most common ones such as:

➤ Vaginal pain
➤ Vaginal odor
➤ Vaginal itching
➤ Loose vagina
➤ Erectile dysfunction
➤ Premature ejaculation
➤ General sexual desire disorder and sexual arousal disorder

Bedroom Justice

> ➢ Peyronie Disease

Men afflicted with Peyronie Disease show signs of depression and withdrawal from their sexual partners. And women with loose Vagina and vaginal pain also withdraw/shy away from sexual activities.

In other to attain optimum dose of sex and receive bedroom justice, one need to be sexually health. Sexual health and wellbeing to be discussed in this chapter as it regards optimum dose of sex includes:

Dyspareunia (painful sexual intercourse)

Interstitial Cystitis – IC

Vaginal Lubrication (eliminate vaginal dryness)

Vaginal Cleanliness (eliminate vaginal odor and itching)

Erectile Dysfunction

Sexual Desire Disorder

Sexual Arousal Disorder

DYSPAREUNIA

Dyspareunia is a Greek word meaning bad sex. Dyspareunia is painful sexual intercourse. The cause of this type of painful sexual intercourse may be of medical, emotional and psychological origin, though sometimes it is often difficult to determine the cause of dyspareunia. This form of sexual intercourse ails both males and females, though it is mainly reported by women. Dyspareunia is a persistent pain in the genitals during sexual intercourse, after sexual intercourse and or before sexual intercourse. The pain causes distraction from pleasure and excitement of sexual intercourse.

Dyspareunia must not be confused with **Vaginismus** which is the involuntary contraction of vaginal muscles and causes severe pain, sometimes far more painful than dyspareunia pains. However, it is noteworthy that vaginismus in women is often preceded by dyspareunia. In women, sometimes vaginal atrophy may be the source of dyspareunia and it is most often seen in postmenopausal women.

For information on Vaginismus, see the books

"The Bedroom Fool" & "The Bedroom Logic"

Symptoms of Dyspareunia in Women

- ➢ Minimal vaginal lubrication
- ➢ Decreased vaginal dilation
- ➢ Vaginal pain during penetration
- ➢ Disappearance and recurrence of pain

Causes of Dyspareunia

The cause of dyspareunia may be natural and or acquired

Natural Causes of Dyspareunia

- ➢ Endometriosis (problem of the uterine cavity and uterine lining that causes recurring pelvic pain, often associated with infertility)
- ➢ Vaginal Septa (natural partition within the vagina. It could be vertical or horizontal)
- ➢ Hypoplasia of the introitus (small vaginal opening)

- Ovarian cysts
- Thickened un-dilatable hymen

Acquired Causes of Dyspareunia Include

Vaginal infection (yeast infection, urinary tract infection, pelvic inflammation disease)

Vulvar vestibulitis (pain in the vulva region)

Tumors (uterine fibroids)

Interstitial Cystitis

Uterine prolapse (for more information on prolapse see the book "The Bedroom Fool")

Genital mutilation

Genital surgery

Dyspareunia in Men

Pain may be experienced by men in the testicular/glans region of the penis following ejaculation or during ejaculation.

Causes Dyspareunia in Men

- Infection of the prostate
- Infection of the bladder
- Infection of the seminal vesicle
- Gonorrhea
- Urethritis – causes pain during genital stimulation
- Prostatitis – causes pain during penile erection/stimulation
- Peyronie's Disease (sometimes caused by circumcision) this can cause pain during sexual arousal and intercourse.

> ➢ Recoil of foreskin – this may cause pain on uncircumcised men, especially if the foreskin is too tight.
> ➢ Another source of pain may be the tear of frenum of the foreskin which often happens during vigorous/intense intercourse.

Treatment of Dyspareunia in Women

If you have any of the symptoms and or signs mentioned above, you may need to consult your doctor.

However, treating vaginal dryness, loose vagina, and elevating estrogen level in the body system may take care of many less serious vaginal problems because most of these problems are inter-related and or is caused because of the presence and or onset of one. For more treatment options see the books

"The Bedroom Fool"

If yours is not serious pain and or condition, some therapy as discussed below may alleviate the situation.

Most pain of dyspareunia as said above disappears over time with little care and therapy.

Removing the source of pain by taking care of the vaginal infection if it is caused by vaginal infection

Talk with your partner to find the best form of caress during intimate sessions.

Practice sessions of caress without penile or finger penetration. This elevates vaginal lubrication and vaginal dilation, which helps in resolving many less serious vaginal ailments.

Oral sex may be helpful, because it also elevates vaginal lubrication and dilation, as the vaginal muscles gets ready for penetration and oozes moisture into the vaginal canal. If the pain is serious, penetration may be avoided during these sessions.

Do not use petroleum jelly and other petroleum derivative products as your vaginal lubricants, because they contain ingredients that will ultimately make the vaginal dry soon after intercourse and or intimate session

Collagen and Elastin supplement may be helpful for bladder muscles and proper bladder functioning

Most other lubricants may not be suitable too

For safety, use vitamin E capsules as your vaginal lubricant. You can also obtain pure grade vitamin E oil in bottle or jar from dealers. Vitamin E is one of the safest and nutrient suitable vaginal lubricants that help to heal the vagina of many short-comings including: vaginal dryness, vaginal atrophy/atrophic vaginitis, loose vagina, itching, etc.

If the pain is experienced more inside the vagina, you may need to discuss with your partner to avoid deep penetration and this could be achieved when the woman lies on her back with her legs extended flat on the bed.

Treatment of Dyspareunia in Men

As discussed above, dyspareunia is mainly caused by prostate infection and prostate health. In this case you may like to engage in therapy and or prevention. If the pain is minimal, you may need to increase consumption of the following foods and mainly calciferous vegetables:

- ➢ Broccoli consumption is good for prostate health.
- ➢ Soy is also beneficial to prostate health.
- ➢ Lycopene in watermelon, tomatoes
- ➢ Goji berries is good for prostate health and prevents prostate cancer.
- ➢ Saw palmetto is good for prostate health and particularly prostate hyperplasia.
- ➢ Collagen and Elastin supplement may be helpful for bladder muscles and proper bladder functioning

For more information see the book "The Bedroom Wisdom"

INSTERSTITIAL CYSTITIS

One of the symptoms of interstitial cystitis is dyspareunia. This disease is characterized by bladder pain during and sometimes after sexual intercourse, and painful urination. In men the pain occurs during and immediately after ejaculation, and also painful urination. The cause is often unknown or idiopathic. Idiopathic is a medical term meaning unknown cause.

Women with interstitial cystitis usually have pain the day following intercourse. They may also experience spasm of the pelvic floor muscle, urinary frequency/urgency.

Treatment for Interstitial Cystitis

The treatment for this disease may be similar to treatment for urinary incontinence. Treatment is mainly made up of physiotherapy including strengthening the pelvic floor muscles.

PEYRONIES DISEASE

Chronic Inflammation of Tunica Albuginea– CITA

This is a man's disease and a disease of the connective tissues, sometimes referred to as a connective tissue disorder. This disease enlists the growth of fibrous plaques (scar tissues – dead cells) in the soft tissue of the penis. This growth may cause pain, abnormal bending of the penis, erectile dysfunction, indentation, thinning and shortening of the penis. It is noteworthy that some men are born with unusually curved penis and such shouldn't be seen as a symptom of peyronie disease. The disease may cause pain during urination and sexual intercourse. It universally affect people of all race but prevalent among the Caucasian population and mainly with men 40years and above. Some studies have also cited members of blood group A to be more susceptible/predisposed to suffer peyronie disease.

Treatment and therapy include: - use of Superoxide Dismutase, Penile extenders, L-arginine, vitamin E, Erectile dysfunction, etc.

URETHRITIS

Urethritis is the inflammation of the urethra and is characterized by pain during urination and general urinary difficulty.

This disease is classified as gonococcal urethritis or non-gonococcal urethritis (NGU). Gonococcal urethritis is caused by Neisseria gonorrhea. And non-gonococcal urethritis is caused by chlamydia trachomatis. This disease afflicts both males and females. Male infection may be detected by whitish discharge from the penis, while it is more difficult to be detected in afflicted females because of possible lack of discharge and other obvious symptoms.

PREVENTION

Practice safe sex by avoiding unprotected sexual activity. Avoid using chemicals that may irritate the urethra including detergents, lotions, spermicides and some contraceptives.

***** *****

BJ

CHAPTER 10

Sexual Desire Disorder
Sexual Arousal Disorder

SEXUAL DYSFUNCTION

SEXUAL MALFUNCTION

Any difficulty arising during any phase or stage of a normal sexual activity is referred to as sexual dysfunction or sexual malfunction. Such difficulty includes:

- ❖ Sexual Desire Disorder
- ❖ Sexual Arousal Disorder
- ❖ Orgasm Disorder - Anorgasmia

Sexual Desire Disorder

Sexual desire disorders sometimes called decreased libido is the absence and or lack of desire for sex, sexual activity, sexual or erotic imagination and fantasies. This may be lack or diminished desire for a particular ones sex partner and or general decreased sexual desire. For a disorder to be qualified as sexual desire disorder, the victim's sexual desire must have been normal and healthy in the past or the victim's sexual desire have always been low or no desire at all.

Sexual desire disorder may be caused by any of the following:

Hormonal Imbalance: Hormonal imbalance such as sudden decrease in estrogen level in a woman's body system and or decrease in man's testosterone level is one of the causes of sexual desire disorder. Decrease in normal level of testosterone in a woman's system may also cause sexual desire disorder.

Hypoactive Sexual Desire Disorder-HSDD

OR Sexual Aversion Disorder

This is the lack and or absence of erotic desire, sexual desire, sexual fantasy and or lack of interest in sexual activity. This disorder must have resulted to distress and interpersonal frictions to be classified as HSDD. This disorder may manifest in forms such as: general lack of or diminished sexual desire, lack of sexual desire for an existing partner, lack of sexual disorder after a life of normal of sexual desire, and lack or diminished sexual desire since birth.

***** *****

***** *****

BJ

CHAPTER 11

ORGASM (Sexual Gratification)

Orgasm is the gratification of all sexual spoiling from sexual desire to sexual arousal through actual sexual intercourse. It is noteworthy that orgasm does not necessarily mean ejaculations, but an intense feeling of relief with the attendant physical and emotional release and surrender to the cellular level of the entire body system. It is the kind of relief and surrender that endures, when you feel you are about to explode with ecstasy: when almost all the cells and tissues of your body system indulge in the said surrender and release of heightened sexual energy in exchange for the ensuing ecstatic explosion.

And that is called Bedroom Justice – Optimum Dose of Sex/Ecstasy.

However, orgasm may be elusive to some people due to some problems which are mostly reversible.

Orgasm Disorders or Anorgasmia

This disorder is called delayed ejaculation in males. Anorgasmia or orgasm disorder is a condition when an individual takes too long to reach and or achieve orgasm or unable to reach and or achieve orgasm even with maximum stimulation. This situation is more common in females than males. This condition may lead to sexual frustration and eventually lack of interest in sex- low sex drive.

The statistics as at the year 2008 shows that about 15% of women have difficulties with orgasm, and 10% of women in the United States alone have never climaxed/had orgasm. And only 29% of women have had and always have orgasms with their partner during sexual intercourse.

While orgasm with men diminished as they age. Women are more likely to understand and achieve regular orgasm as they age.

Causes of Orgasm disorder include:

- ✓ The use of antidepressants
- ✓ Psychiatric disorder
- ✓ Diabetic neuropathy
- ✓ Multiple sclerosis
- ✓ Genital mutilation (including female circumcision and vaginal reconstructive surgery)
- ✓ Pelvic trauma – from wounds in the pelvic region
- ✓ Hormonal Imbalance
- ✓ Hysterectomy
- ✓ Spinal cord Injury
- ✓ Drug (opiate) addiction

Causes of anorgasmia (orgasm disorder) differ with type of anorgasmia.

Bedroom Justice

Types of Anorgasmia

Primary Anorgasmia

A person with primary anorgasmia has never experienced orgasm. Primary anorgasmia is more prevalent in women than in men. This type of anorgasmia only occurs in men who do not have bulb-cavernous reflex. Women victims of primary anorgasmia are not easily aroused sexually and receive very little sexual excitement. Due to lack of release of orgasmic energy after stimulation and engorgement of the genitals, they often suffer from sexual frustration, restlessness, and pelvic pain.

Sexual repression due to culture and or religion has been touted as possible causes of women primary anorgasmia.

Male primary anorgasmia may be caused by circumcision. As men get older, the ability to reach orgasm diminishes. Remember the mere fact that a man ejaculates does not mean he reached or achieved orgasm.

Secondary Anorgasmia

A person suffering from secondary anorgasmia is a person who have been having orgasm but for one reason or the other losses the ability to achieve orgasm over time. Men and women have about equal chances of suffering from secondary anorgasmia.

Causes of secondary anorgasmia include:

- ➢ Alcoholism
- ➢ Depression

➢ Grief

➢ Surgery – Chiefly hysterectomy

➢ Vaginal reconstructive Surgery (vaginoplasty)

➢ Decrease or lack of Estrogen

➢ Psychological injury and trauma such as "rape"

➢ Prostate cancer and prostatectomy

Situational Anorgasmia

This is a situation whereby a person achieves orgasm in one situation and not in another. The situation may be the type of sexual stimulation, different partners, certain conditions, duration and intensity of foreplay.

Random Anorgasmia

This is a situation where one has not had orgasm enough, on a regular or near regular basis to be able to establish the desirability of orgasm.

***** *****

PART 5

VAGINAL MUSCLE EXERCISE

***** *****

BJ

CHAPTER 12

VAGINAL TIGHTENING

Through the pages and chapters of this book to this point, we will assume that we have determined that the basic due process for bedroom justice is in place. Now you need to check the conditions of your vaginal muscles to make sure you can put them to use for an earth-shattering orgasm – earth-shattering bedroom justice. A tight, elastic and lubricated vagina makes a man and the woman feel the ecstasy of every inch of his travel down the pleasure mine between the woman's legs. It is the most essential component of the magic of a come-back exploration – daily justice in the bedroom. For the most part, a strong, toned and controllable vaginal muscle is associated with tight and rejuvenated vagina. Strengthening your vaginal wall muscle and your love muscle (pc muscles) is essential in controlling and making the best of bedroom plea to achieve the desired justice – intensified orgasm. We will discuss measures to tighten and strengthen the pelvic floor muscles, PC muscle, and vaginal wall muscle, improve orgasm and empower your sex life.

It is also good to know at this point that achieving orgasm is dependent on the contraction of the love muscles (pc muscles). In other to have orgasm under any circumstance, the PC muscle needs to contract, and that is what makes orgasm possible. When the PC muscle is relaxed, flabby and unable to contract, then orgasm is impossible. The PC muscle is a member of the pelvic floor muscles. When the PC muscle is flabby and weak, most other muscles are weak and flabby to the same and or varying degree. Lack of orgasm therefore is a sign of weak vaginal muscles, weak pc muscles and the associated loose vagina. Optimal PC muscles will make it possible for you to be able to hold and squeeze or clamp and clench his penis as he travels up and down your vaginal canal. As you clamp

and clench the penis with your vaginal wall muscles or pc

muscles, you can massage it quickly and or slowly and release it

at will. Like this you can control both your and his orgasm and

achieve the optimum dose of sexual intercourse for the desired

bedroom justice.

Ways by which the PC muscle, vaginal wall muscles, and the vagina could be tightened includes:

❖ Vagina Muscle Exercise

❖ Vagina Tightening Creams and Sprays

❖ Vagina Rejuvenation Procedure

❖ Hormone Replacement

❖ Food for Vagina Tightening and General Wellbeing

❖ Vaginal Herbal Remedies

For the purpose of this book, we will only discuss vaginal muscle exercise.

For more information on Vaginal Tightening Creams and Sprays: Vaginal Rejuvenation Procedure: Hormone Replacement: Food For Vaginal Tightening and General Vaginal wellbeing: Vaginal Herbal Remedies,

You Need To See The Book "The Bedroom Fool". The **S**ecret to tightening, elasticizing and rejuvenating your vagina is well laid out in the guide called "The Bedroom Fool".

VAGINAL MUSCLE EXERCISE

Vaginal muscle exercise(s) is the easiest and least expensive way to tone, and condition the vaginal wall muscle, and tighten the vaginal opening and vaginal canal. To reap the benefits of these exercises you need to be patient and religiously follow the steps involved in the stages of the exercise. In tightening your vaginal wall muscle and PC muscle you will improve your orgasm, making orgasm as strong, intense and satisfying as you never thought possible, have quality sex and generally enhance, empower and re-ignite your sex life and that of your sex partner. Vaginal muscle exercise could be done at anytime and anywhere and it is not strenuous. Some women prefer the medical and or surgical procedures that cost thousands of dollars for reasons that may range from immediate result to being ill informed. Good thing about vaginal muscle exercises is that they do not cause any harm to the body and they are very affordable and within the reach of every woman who desires to have a tight vagina, improved sex life and enhanced and intense orgasm. The impediment to the fruitful result of these vaginal exercises is that most women would not have the will power and endurance to continue doing them until they get results. If done regularly and correctly they often work, and work abundantly.

When your vaginal muscles are well exercised, the vaginal walls become tight thus improving the texture and feel of the vagina to the penis. You have more control of the movement of the vagina muscles during intercourse, so much so that you can clamp and clench his penis at will. You can squeeze, massage, ease and release his penis quickly and at will, and in so doing control his and your orgasm. The early post-virgin "click" associated with penis pull-out could be attributed to the natural strong, tight and elastic teenage vagina muscle, after discounting vaginal flatulence. You can reclaim this power and glory by simple vaginal muscle exercise.

KEGEL EXERCISE

Kegel Exercise is attributed to Dr. Arnold Kegel who discovered the simple exercise. In the 1940's Dr. Kegel found out that one can actually tighten the vagina and strengthen the vaginal muscles by exercising the PC muscle and pelvic floor muscles. The simple squeeze-and-hold vaginal exercises specifically designed to target pelvic floor strengthening then become known as **Kegels**.

Bedroom Justice

Kegel exercises have long been accepted as one of the best method to tighten your PC muscle and vagina.

Kegels is good for women of all ages. It is often advisable when one starts at a young age to do Kegels. The first thing to be done when starting Kegels is to identify the right muscle to be exercised and toned. This is good because it is very easy to bring other, irrelevant muscles into play while doing Kegels. To isolate the pelvic muscle and target the right muscle, you must:

- ✓ not pull in your tummy
- ✓ not squeeze your legs together
- ✓ not tighten your buttocks
- ✓ not hold your breath

Remember the sensation you feel when you have to use the washroom/bathroom to urinate, and how you suck it in and hold it. The very muscle you use to hold back the urine is the relevant muscle. This is a Kegel. Now pretend that you have to use the washroom desperately, now contract your relevant muscles to hold it. Did you do it right? If so, that is Kegels and you can do Kegels whenever you want and wherever you are. They are one of the best exercises you need to do if you want to make your vaginal muscles stronger and your vagina tighter.

Now let's do the real one. Do you have the urge to urinate? Yes? Good. Go to the washroom and let the tap (urine) on. Now stop the flow of urine. Hold it! Now let go, let urine flow again. Hold it again. Hold! Now let flow again.

Bedroom Justice

The muscle you use to hold the urine flow is the PC muscle you need to exercise and tone. Provided you did not pull your stomach muscles, squeeze your legs together, tighten your buttocks and or hold your breath Remember, don't do this often, it is not safe as an exercise during urinary urge.

To further identify the PC Muscle, do the following:

Sit on a clean toilet and spread your legs as wide as you can, then urinate and empty your bladder completely. Insert a finger into the vagina and contract the same muscle as if you want to stop the flow of urine, feel the contractions.

Step 1

Squeeze and hold the PC muscle for 4 seconds. Relax and repeat the process.

Step 2

Contract and release the PC muscle about 10 to 12 times.

Step 3

Contract the PC muscle and hold for 10 to 15 seconds.

This is somewhat how Kegels work. However, for comprehensive details, you should read more literature on Kegel exercises. You need to do this as many times as possible every day. On the average do 20 sessions of 10 contraction, totaling 200 or 300 as the case may be.

Remember, the result is never immediate; you need to be patient and persistent. Sometimes it takes at least a couple of weeks if not months for the result to manifest. And you will be able to enjoy intense orgasm, clamp, and clench and massage your partner's penis and enslave him sexually. Motivation and determination are the very key for success with Kegels. Exercises provide resistance. Remember just like ordinary exercise, going to the gym, you do not see any tangible result in the first week or two, you need to continue going to the gym until you tone your body muscles and achieve the desired body tone and shape, the same applies to Kegels and your PC muscle. Because Kegels is an invisible exercise that can be done anywhere, whether you're alone, talking to a friend, or in a crowd of people, in a grocery store and in the subway, etc., does not make it any different from any other exercise.

In an effort to perfect and or make Kegel exercises more effective, devices, objects and methods have been designed to aid in Kegels.

Some Kegel devices include:

> ➢ Kegel Balls
> ➢ Jade eggs
> ➢ Duotone Balls
> ➢ Smart Balls
> ➢ Pleasure Balls
> ➢ Vaginal Cones

The balls and cones differ in sizes and weight. They have small, medium and large sizes and weight categories. The one you use as a person depends on your size, and stage in the exercise.

They can be made from metal, plastic, stone, marble, ceramic and silicone. Balls made from metal, ceramics and stone are somewhat safer as they do not absorb bacteria. The balls are sterilized before using. You can sterilize the balls using hot water or steam. Balls and cones made of plastic are often light in weight and need to be made heavier with some added weights inside the balls. Metal balls are hollow balls and may also contain ball bearings inside for added weight. Silicone and rubber balls are soft and can be squeezed to acquire added resistance. When you insert the Kegel balls into the vagina, you need to contract the PC muscles to hold them in place. The movement of the PC muscles can also move the balls back and forth while sitting down, this in itself may provide some form of arousal or stimulation for some women. However, a beginner may want to start off with large balls as they are easier to grasp and hold with the PC muscle.

While standing, insert the ball into the vagina and squeeze/contract the PC muscle to hold it in place. Try holding the ball for say ten seconds. Then repeat the exercise ten to 30 times a day, giving a total of 200 to 300 contractions. It is very important to do the exercises daily to achieve results. After your muscles have improved, you can move on to smaller balls, which are a little more difficult to hold and needs experienced muscle to hold them.

POSITION TO EMPLOY WHILE EXERCISING WITH KEGEL BALLS AND DEVICES

You can use the balls to exercise in different positions including:

Sitting

In this position, open your legs and insert the ball. Close your legs and start to use the same muscle you use to hold the flow of urine to try and move the ball inside you back and forth for as many times as you could. Do sessions per day

Standing

Insert the ball inside your vaginal canal and close your legs and try to hold the ball from falling. Hold as long as you can, relax the muscle and contract again. Do this session as many times as you can per day. Try doing it with your legs open and then wide open and see if you can hold the ball in place.

Squatting

While squatting with legs wide open, insert the ball into the vagina and use your vaginal muscles to push the ball inner into your vaginal canal. Repeat as many times as possible.

CONES

Most vaginal cones are made of stainless steel, marble and ceramics and most vaginal cones have the shape of a regular tampon. Vaginal cones also come in different sizes and weights. Cones are better employed in Kegels while standing.

OTHER METHODS

ELECTRICAL STIMULATION

This is sometimes called Neuroelectrical stimulation. A probe of this device inserted into the pelvic floor generates electric current which contracts and relaxes the vaginal muscle.

NEOCONTROL

This method employs a chair which generates a magnetic field that stimulates the pelvic floor.

OTHER EXERCISES FOR THE PELVIC FLOOR MUSCLES

What is the Pelvic Floor?

The pelvic floor is that point in the pelvic region of the body where all the connective tissues and muscles that support all the organs of the pelvis connect. And the pelvic floor muscles are the muscles that are connected to the pelvic floor. Some of the muscles include:

➢ Vaginal muscle
➢ Rectal Muscle
➢ Urethra
➢ Uterus
➢ Perineum muscle

PERINEAL MASSAGE

The name given to this exercise arises from the perineum, which as seen from the topical body, is the skin that connects/between the rectum and the vagina. From the inside, the perineal body stretches inwards from the perineum area and provides the insertion point/base of the other muscles (eight muscles) that forms the pelvic floor. When the perineum is massaged, blood circulation is increased, and more blood flows to the pelvic floor improving the health of the pelvic floor muscles.

To massage the perineum, you insert oiled thumbs into the base of the vaginal opening and press downwards towards the back/spine. Do this as many times a week as you can. This massage improves the flexibility or elasticity of the pelvic floor muscles. Perineal massage involves lubricating the thumbs and inserting them inside the base of the vagina, then exerting downward pressure toward the back of the spine. A person's tolerance will increase as she practices, and the pelvic floor will become more flexible. This can be done by any woman seeking to improve pelvic floor flexibility. Perineal massage is especially good for pregnant women because it combines breathing with downward pressure thereby improving flexibility, which is particularly helpful during birth.

SQUATTING EXERCISE

This exercise is easy. You can squat as many times and many sessions as you can per day. It helps to strengthen the pelvic floor and the pelvic floor muscles. Squatting is good for women of all ages.

***** *****

***** *****

PART 6

NEUROTRANSMITTERS

ENDORPHINS

VASODILATORS

***** *****

BJ

CHAPTER 13

Neurotransmitters

Endorphins

Vasodilators

Throughout the chapters and pages of this book, we discussed topics ranging from attraction, law of contagion, chemical attraction, pheromones, positive mental attitude, and sympathetic science through sexual desire, libido, sexual health and wellbeing, orgasm, to vaginal muscle exercise.

In all the topics, all effort is towards an optimal condition and environment for the inducement and secretion of biochemicals into the Central Nervous System (CNS), Peripheral Nervous System (PNS) and the brain to activate the final gratification (orgasm) of all sexual endeavors. The said bio-chemicals help to give the body a natural sexual high in preparation for love making and sex. The said bio-chemicals are neuro-chemicals, neurotransmitters, endorphins, anticholinergenics, vaso-dilators and hormones could be explained as follows:

NEUROTRANSMITTERS

Neurotransmitters are chemical messengers that relay the messages sent from the brain through the nervous system to the point of action of the said message or command.

In the absence of these chemical messengers, messages and commands may not be relayed and most human actions and emotions cannot be expressed.

Few examples of neurotransmitters as it regards optimum dose of sex and Bedroom Justice are as follows: norepinephrine, acetylcholine, serotonin, and dopamine. Some of the neurotransmitters regulate sex drive, libido, stress, sleep and even hormonal levels in the body system.

FUNTIONS:

Acetylcholine – controls the action of involuntary movements of smooth muscles including pc muscles (all genital muscles – vaginal, penile muscles). It regulates and controls orgasm and ejaculation. During intercourse and orgasm, the smooth muscles of the genitals contracts involuntarily for orgasm to happen.

Anticholinergenic, (example, elemicin) blocks the action of neurotransmitters (such as acetylcholine) in the both the Central Nervous System (CNS – Brain + Spinal cord) and the Peripheral Nervous system (blood vessels and nerves besides brain and spinal cord) from binding to its receptor nerves cells/fibers. The nerve fibers of the parasympathetic system are responsible for the involuntary movements of smooth muscles present in body such as: Urinary tract/bladder, pelvic floor muscles, genital muscles, lungs, etc.

Anticholinergenics are divided into three categories to represent their targets in the central and/or peripheral nervous system: antimuscarinic agents, ganglionic blockers, and neuromuscular blockers. Neuromuscular blockers could be useful in treating urinary incontinence.

Other examples of anticholinergenics include: atropine and dicycloverine.

The Anticholinergenic effect of say **Elemicin** (elemicin is a phenylpropene - a natural organic anticholinergic compound) prolongs and helps you to control the contraction of the PC/genital muscles and thus prolongs stamina and intensifies orgasm.

Oxytocin – works as a hormone (outside the brain) and neurotransmitter (within the brain), often called the love hormone. Oxytocin induces, enhances and intensifies orgasm. Oxytocin hinders the release of hormones responsible for stress known as cortisol, and also reduces blood pressures that occur due to anxiety.

In men, oxytocin helps to establish quick emotional bonding and desire. While in women, quick emotional bonding, desire and multiple orgasms is especially enhanced.

Dopamine and norepinephrine regulates libido/sexual desire/sexual arousal

Dopamine – produce feel-good mood and regulates stress by reducing levels of cortisol

GABA –gama-aminobutyric acid – directly regulates smooth muscle tone including vaginal, pc muscles and penile muscles.

Serotonin – regulates sleep, mood-boosting and relaxation

Histamine is released as a neurotransmitter in the brain.

Histamine is excellent in aiding erection, sexual arousal and orgasm in both men and women. Folate - Vitamin B9-folic acid helps to enhance the reach of orgasm in both male and female, because it aids in the release of histamine. Hesperidin in combination with Vitamin C helps to maintain the health of genital muscles especially the collagen and elastic linings of the vaginal canal.

There are known foods, drinks and vitamins that contain and or enhance the inducement and secretion of neurotransmitters into the nervous system.

For More Information on foods, vitamins and minerals that are rich in and or enhance the inducement and secretion of neurotransmitters,

See the Books:

Bedroom Logic

Bedroom Wisdom

The Bedroom Fool

ENDORPHINS

Endorphins which mean endogenous morphine is endogenous opioid peptides that mimic the actions of neurotransmitters, and as such functions as neurotransmitters. Endorphins are produced in the pituitary and the hypothalamus during exercise, pain (for comfort or reduction of pain), love, orgasm or when you consume something good or spicy.

Endorphins produce analgesia and general feeling of well-being and mood boosting.

Endorphins are the bio-chemicals that are triggered or secreted during kissing, love making, sex, and increases the feelings of attraction between two people.

Endorphins help to give the body a natural sexual high in preparation for love making and sex.

Exercise induces the release of endorphins and also wards off depression. Some exercise has been touted to induce labour

Myristicin belongs to the class of monoamine oxidase inhibitors (MAOIs). Monoamine oxidase inhibitors are a class of antidepressant drugs, used in the treatment of atypical/unusual/light depression. This is what provides the euphoria and feel good mood. Myristicin is responsible for the euphoria and the hallucination.

VASODILATION & VASO-DILATORS

Vasodilation means to dilate (make wider) the blood vessel and in so doing causes greater and adequate circulation/flow of blood in the body system, including greater and adequate blood supply to the genitals, inducing sexual arousal, sex drive and libido.

Better blood flow to the genitals, creates greater arousal for men and women. Adequate blood supply to the genitals is good for sexual desire and sexual arousal.

Examples of Vasodilators are as follows:

Nitric oxide is a gas molecule which helps to open the potassium channel, which causes the blood vessels to relax – vasodilation, and this aids the proper blood circulation and blood supply to the genitals. Adequate blood supply to the genitals aids sexual arousal, sexual desire, sex drive, and libido.

Magnesium helps dilate blood vessels. Vaso-dilation improves blood circulation including the supply of blood to the genitals.

Potassium – Helps for the proper functioning of the muscles and is very essential in relaxing the blood vessels – Vasodilation, and encourages healthy blood circulation in the vessels and capillaries. Potassium activates nitric oxide, which relaxes the arteries, reducing the pressure on the arteries and encourages optimal flow and circulation of blood. In so doing, potassium aids in supplying adequate nutrients to the genitals. Potassium is also very essential for the proper functioning of the thyroid.

Bedroom Justice

Theobromine is a myocardial stimulant as well as a vasodilator. It increases heartbeat, but also dilates blood vessels, causing a reduced blood pressure. In so doing it encourages healthy blood circulation and aids the supply of blood to the genitals, a good feature of healthy sex drive and libido.

L-arginine induces the release of nitric oxide in the body system. Nitric oxide is a gas molecule that help smooth muscle in arterioles dilate and relax (vasodilation), thereby increasing blood flow and circulation in the body system. And this includes adequate blood supply to the genitals which will induce or trigger sexual desire, and sexual arousal.

Proanthocyanidins are vasoactive polyphenols: meaning that they act on blood vessels. Proanthocyanidins suppress production of a protein endothelin-1 that constricts blood vessels. By working against vaso-constriction, proanthocyanidins are vasodilators. Proanthocyanidins induces and optimize the production of nitric oxide in the artery walls relaxing them and reduced pressure thus allowing greater and adequate blood flow and circulation in the body system, including adequate blood supply to the genitals.

For more information on foods, vegetables, supplements, vitamins and most importantly on How to Mix and match foods , vitamins, enzymes and supplement to produce the desired result and provide Optimum Dose of Sex – Bedroom Justice:

See the Book – <u>Bedroom Wisdom</u>

Bedroom Justice

In <u>Bedroom Wisdom</u> you will find lots of reasons and explanations why for example it is advisable to eat say:

1. Banana in combination with peanuts and a cup of mixture of fresh watermelon + pineapple juice. You recall, people have been doing this, may be without knowing why and as such will not know at what time it is most pertinent and applicable.

2. What watermelon juice or pineapple juice can do for you hours and minutes before sexual session(s).

3. Why and how Dark chocolate helps to boost and attain optimum dose of sex and is as well a known vasodilator.

And why mixing and matching some vitamins and foods could be reducing blood pressure and atherosclerosis. Why some foods are used as aphrodisiacs.

4. You will also learn how to use <u>collagen and elastin to strengthen vaginal muscles</u> and <u>aid penile erection</u>.

5. How vitamin B6, oxytocin, and vitamin B9 (folate or folic acid) can intensify orgasm and your dose of sex.

How vitamin B9, Zinc, Selenium, could improve sperm motility, sperm viability and virility. How selenium and vitamin B9 could improve the quality and health of the ova and general fertility.

***** *****

***** *****

BJ

CHAPTER 14

Innate Style

Sex Accessories (optional)

Intervals

Every individual has a particular sexual position(s) that triggers the most sexual feeling, sexual arousal and enhances orgasm. This is one of those acts of sexual activity that is entirely personal and seems to have no known determinants. The only clue as regards sexual positions and sexual excitement and orgasm enhancement is only that certain position makes vaginal penetration deeper. And other positions may bring the scrotal sac in better contact with the vulva, vaginal orifice and or make the penile shaft touch the edge of the clitoral area during the normal thrusting movement. The choice of using sexual toys and accessories is also personal and optional. However, it has been established that sexually healthy individuals who has healthy libido, stamina, and who engages the information laid out in the books under bedroom Politics series rarely need toys and accessories as supplemental aid to go to paradise. They can always achieve optimum dose of sex on their own using simple knowledge obtained from foods, fruits, vegetables, vitamins, supplements and general sex regimen.

At other times, people use toys and accessories to achieve erection and arousal. Some of the common accessories include:

➤ Clitoral vacuum pump – to improve blood flow to the clitoris, genitals, improve sensation, improve sexual arousal

➤ Penis pump - to achieve penile erection

There are more modern toys and sex accessories in the market today.

Intervals

Sometimes it is said that healthy intervals between sexual sessions is also a factor to achieving optimum dose of sex and bedroom justice. However, the interval between sexual sessions is better established by the parties involved, because every person(s) have different rate of replenishment of hormonal levels, stamina, sex drive and libido.

***** *****

***** *****

The End

Bedroom Justice

GENERAL BRIEF

It is a well-known fact albeit unspoken fact that the only logical justice in the bedroom is healthy and vibrant sex drive, sexual desire, sexual arousal, libido and ultimately sexual intercourse and sexual gratification - orgasm. In the general politics of any relationship, and marriage, the politics of the bedroom is the most essential and in this, Bedroom Justice – Optimum Dose of Sex is most vital.

Guess Why?

Because once you and your sex partner are happy each time you hop aboard the wagon on your journey to heaven, to paradise, the rest of the drag that is existential in any relationship becomes more manageable. And as you see from what you read so far from the pages of this book, that mere sexual intercourse and ejaculation(s) does not necessarily mean orgasm.

Orgasm is rather an intense feeling of relief with the attendant physical and emotional release and surrender to the cellular level of the entire body system. It is the kind of relief and surrender that endures, when you feel you are about to explode with ecstasy: when almost all the cells and tissues of your body system indulge in the said surrender and release of heightened sexual energy in exchange for the ensuing ecstatic explosion.

<u>And that is called Bedroom Justice – Optimum Dose of Sex/Ecstasy.</u>

***** *****

Bedroom Justice

GLOSSARY OF TERMS

Anorgasmia – sexual arousal disorder where the person takes unusually long time to achieve orgasm or unable to achieve orgasm

Asexuality - lack of sexual attraction towards other people irrespective of gender

Sexual desire disorder – a disease or ailment that prevents an individual from having sexual desire

Sexual arousal disorder – a disease or ailment that prevents an individual from having sexual arousal

Vaginal muscles – the muscles (flesh) lining the vaginal canal

Stratified – having layers, not a solid whole

Epithelial – membranous tissues of one or more layers of cells, always having protective or covering functions.

Nervi Erigentis – The nerve responsible for penile erection

Anterior wall – front wall

Posterior wall – back wall

Vaginal canal – the hole inside the vagina

Sub-mucosa – under the mucosa

Vomeronasal organ - chemosensory organ located at the base of the nasal septum

Sympathetic Science/Logic - science or invocative practice based on imitation, repeat/recall and or correspondence

Endorphins - love or feel-good brain chemicals

Emotional stimuli– emotional stimulation

Bedroom Justice

Elastin – structural protein

Frigidity – a type of sexual arousal dysfunction, you may say a woman's version of erectile dysfunction

Vaginal muscularis – vaginal smooth muscles

PC muscle – Pelvic muscle (aka Love muscle)

Estrogen – female sex hormone (also present in men in smaller quantity)

Progesterone – male sex hormone (also present in female in smaller quantity)

Testosterone – the sex drive or libido hormone. It helps give the male characteristics

Incontinence - inability to stop urine leakage from the bladder, the loss of control over the muscle that controls the bladder opening and closure

Latent Homosexuality – Unexpressed, never expressed or suppressed homosexuality in an individual

Menopause – the phase when a woman stops seeing her menstrual cycle, stop ovulating.

Premenopause – phase before menopause. It is also called perimenopause

Vaginal atrophy – the thinning and wasting away of the vaginal wall

Vasodilation - dilation or increase in the diameter of blood vessels

Vasoconstriction–Constriction or reduction in the size of the diameter of blood vessels

Bedroom Justice

Structural changes – changes in the structure, shape, form

Bladder – the human urine sac

Bladder muscle – the muscle that controls the opening and closing of the bladder for the passage of urine

Rectal wall muscles – the muscles lining the rectal canal

Rectum – the tube through which stool is pushed out to the outside as you defecate

Vaginal Prolapse – vaginal collapse, when all the muscles became loose, and the bladder or rectum falls into the vaginal canal

Flatulence – outing of air

Vaginal Flatulence – expelling air from the vagina (vaginal farting)

Pleasure tunnel – vaginal canal

Pleasure mine – vaginal canal

Kegels – name given to vaginal wall muscle exercise as an attribute to Dr. Kegel who developed/discovered the exercise in the 1940's

Kegel Exercise - name given to vaginal wall muscle and PC muscle exercise as an attribute to Dr. Kegel who developed/discovered the exercise in the 1940's

Kegel balls – Devices and objects developed over the years to help target the exact PC muscle as you perform Kegels

Pelvic Floor - The pelvic floor is that point in the pelvic region of the body where all the connective tissues and muscles that support all the organs of the pelvis connects

Hormones – Bio-chemicals (chemicals of the body) in the body system that affects body changes and functions

Hormonal changes – changes in the levels of the body hormones

Sexual addiction - uncontrollable sexual outbursts, sexual behaviors and sexual thoughts

Stinging Wasp – an insect

Symptom – manifested sign

Phytoestrogen – estrogens that are naturally present in plants

Estrogen-like chemicals – chemicals that resemble estrogen

Estrogenic activities – activities native to estrogens

Neurotransmitters – chemical messenger/body electrical transmitters

Omega-3 fatty acids – they are not acids in the common sense of the word acid. It is the name given to some essential fats that is good for the body system

Polyunsaturated Amino acids- long/multiple chain unsaturated amino acids

Monounsaturated amino acids – one chain unsaturated amino acid

Optimum hormonal level – perfect level for the body estrogen, a level at which it is at its best

Hormonal imbalance – imbalance of the levels of the hormones in the body system

Muscular contraction and relaxation – the ease and squeeze actions/movements of the body muscles

Roe – Fish eggs harvested for food (often unfertilized eggs)

Sperm Count – The quantity and quality of sperm – semen volume

Sperm Motility – The agility or mobility of sperm, ability to move towards the Ova to fertilize it

Banana Corm – Base stem of the banana plant

***** *****

***** *****

ABOUT BE YOUR DREAM PRESS

Be Your Dream Press is an imprint of Obrake USA LLC. We are publishers of non-fiction books. Books published by Be Your Dream Press are mainly books that help people to be whatever they want to be. Books that help people succeed in doing whatever legitimate thing they want to engage in.

Be Your Dream Press publishes series of health and beauty books, women health books and the very popular series called Financial Democracy Series.

Books by Be Your Dream Books Include:
- ➢ Bedroom Wisdom
- ➢ Bedroom Logic
- ➢ Bedroom Fool
- ➢ Secrets To Skin Glow and Radiance
- ➢ Secrets To Hair Growth and Sheen

FINANCIAL DEMOCRACY SERIES
- ❖ A Manufacturer without A Factory
- ❖ Steps to Sell, Supply and Do Business with New York City
- ❖ Steps to Sell, Supply and Do Business with Large Corporations in USA
- ❖ Steps to Sell, Supply and Do Business with Educational Institutions in USA
- ❖ Steps to Sell, Supply and Do Business with International Institutions and Organizations
- ❖ Dozen Businesses You Can Start and Run in USA

For more information visit us at:

www.obrake.com/books

OTHER BOOKS BY Be Your Dream Press

FINANCIAL DEMOCRACY SERIES – CANADA

➢ Two Dozen Businesses You Can Start and Run in Canada

➢ No Canadian Experience

FINANCIAL DEMOCRACY SERIES – SOUTH AFRICA

❖ Steps to Sell, Supply and Do Business with National, Provincial, Local and Municipal Government of South Africa

❖ Steps to Sell, Supply and Do Business with Public and Private Corporations in South Africa

❖ How to Start and Run Your Business in South Africa

❖ Two Dozen Businesses You Can Start and Run in South Africa

❖ When South African Banks Say No

Visit us at: www.obrake.com

***** *****

BEDROOM JUSTICE: Optimum Dose of Sex

It is a well-known fact albeit unspoken fact that the only logical justice in the bedroom is healthy and vibrant sex drive, sexual desire, sexual arousal, libido and ultimately sexual intercourse and sexual gratification - orgasm. In the general politics of any relationship, and marriage, the politics of the bedroom is the most essential and in this, Bedroom Justice – Optimum Dose of Sex is most vital. Guess Why? Because once you and your sex partner are happy each time you hop aboard the wagon on your journey to heaven, to paradise, the rest of the drag that is existential in any relationship becomes manageable. And as you will learn from the pages of this book, mere sexual intercourse and ejaculation(s) does not necessarily mean orgasm and Optimum Dose of Sex. Orgasm is rather an intense feeling of relief with the attendant physical and emotional release and surrender to the cellular level of the entire body system. It is the kind of relief and surrender that endures, when you feel you are about to explode with ecstasy: when almost all the cells and tissues of your body system indulges in the said surrender to sexual energy in exchange for the ensuing ecstatic explosion.

And it's called Bedroom Justice – Optimum Dose of Sex

In This Edition You Will Find:

- ➢ How to Optimize Your Sex Life
- ➢ Employ Sympathetic Science for Orgasmic Experiences
- ➢ Intensify Orgasm with Natural Enzymes and Endorphins
- ➢ Revive Your Sexual Energy with Vitamins and Supplements

BE YOUR DREAM PRESS

www.obrake.com

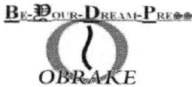

Be-Your-Dream-Press
OBRAKE

www.ingramcontent.com/pod-product-compliance
Lightning Source LLC
Chambersburg PA
CBHW020006290326
41935CB00007B/320